Pain in the Wreck

Whiplash Trauma from a Motor Vehicle Accident?

What you do in the next 14 days determines how your hidden injuries will impact your entire life. By following these simple steps will get you back to normal in the least amount of time with the lowest cost possible!

Dr. Alan Khiger

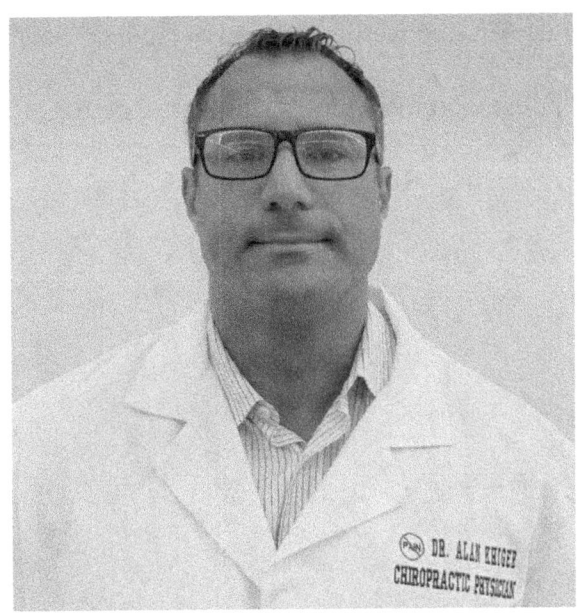

Dr. Alan Khiger | Amazing Spine Care

Dr. Alan Khiger is a graduate of Life University, School of Chiropractic

Medicine, Atlanta, GA, Licensed Doctor of Chiropractic Medicine in

Florida, and has worked in this capacity

in personal injury, workers comp and cash practice patients for the past

six years. Also certified by the American College of Addictionology in

Auricular therapy for patients who

develop substance abuse disorder, Dr. Khiger's specialties include

working with the elderly, children, and new/pregnant mothers.

He has held professional positions in both specialty and general practice

chiropractic care, one of his favorite specialties is that of neuro-

musculoskeletal disorders.

Dr. Khiger is a healer, and well versed in how to help people find alignment and holistic bodily health. In addition, he fluently speaks three languages: Spanish, Russian, and English.

Learn More: www.AmazingSpineCare.com

Contents

Interview with Dr. Alan Khiger

~ *Dr. Khiger, go ahead and tell us about Amazing Spine Care.*

Dr. Alan Khiger: Amazing Spine Care is a clinic that manages whiplash trauma from the car accidents, and also chronic pain, patients that have chronic neuromuscular skeletal conditions, and we'll be also working out with the population who are fighting addiction and substance abuse as well.

~ *You're typically working with people that have had some type of accident, like a car accident. Is that the focus of your practice?*

Dr. Alan Khiger: Yeah, primarily focused on the motor vehicle trauma at our clinic.

Dr. Alan Khiger

~ ***Why specifically car accidents? Is that something that typically someone would have a greater need for chiropractic care than other types of trauma?***

Dr. Alan Khiger: Yeah. In today's world, there's a lot of whiplash conditions that occur during the car accidents and they go misdiagnosed, mismanaged, what have you, and the population is still suffering for a great deal of time to overcome those injuries. They don't have a clear idea how to get through these injuries or who to contact when this is occurring.

~ ***You mentioned whiplash, and I think that's a term that a lot of people hear about, and might be a little bit confused as far as what exactly that it is. What are some of the things that people should be concerned with as far as symptoms to make sure that they realize that this is something to definitely get taken care of regarding whiplash?***

Dr. Alan Khiger: First and foremost, they can experience headaches, pain in the neck, pain in the mid-back, pain in the lower back, numbness and tingling in the hands and feet. 50% of patients suffer concussions such as that that occur on the football field. They can also suffer pain in their arms, wrist depending on what position they are at the time of the accident and where the hands and the feet will place. For example, if it's on the gas pedal or near the dashboard, they can bruise their knee.

Also some of the severe cases where, of course, there can be lacerations of the organs which is called the visceral conditions where someone can wind up with a broken rib. Then, the rib punctures the lung, or kidney, what have you. The patient may have more severe disorders such as blood in their stool or difficulty breathing, and chronic pain in the chest and back as well.

~ *I think that sometimes people that get in a car accident might feel like, "I was in an accident. I can wait a while to go get seen." What happens if they wait even a few weeks to see if they can deal with the pain?*

Dr. Alan Khiger: The problem is going to get worse if they wait because they're basically thinking that, "Okay, I went to the gym and I can have the same type of injury that I got while working out at the gym. It's probably just pain and a strain. I'll just use ice, take some ibuprofen, it will go away," but unfortunately, that's not the case because you have a lot more structures in the body that's involved during the accident.

That's what makes this process complicated and painful for the patient because once you have cellular body organs and body tissues that are signaling your brain that your body is in need of repair, then the condition gets a lot more chronic, and it gets a lot more painful over time since nobody is addressing it. The body has a self-healing mechanism that's basically telling you, "Go ahead, do something about it because I need to be repaired. I need to be fixed."

~   *I think that it's really interesting how the body works with these signals and I can only imagine that there may even be hidden injuries that you might feel a pain in one spot but you could get in there and discover hidden injuries. What are some of the significance*

of how hidden injuries impact the overall recovery?

Dr. Alan Khiger: For example, the patient can have an alteration in their spine. In other words, the spine went out of alignment when the patient got ambushed by a car. While the patient can walk around thinking, "Okay, I have something going on but it's not really that much of a bother to me. I am actually able to do things that I was prior to the accident but now, I am doing it with somewhat difficulty. I have a little bit loss of sleep. I sometimes wake up once or twice at night."

Then, you take the x-ray, and you're looking at this patient's spine, it looks like a leaning tower that's about to be collapsed once you put a little push on it. Then, the patient will see the x-ray and he's completely shocked, "Oh my. This is me. This is how I am walking around." "Yeah, this is you walking around because you might not have a symptom as a result of this collision that you've had but if you go unnoticed for some amount of time, this is going to get worse, and this is basically a time bomb waiting to explode in your body."

~	*Isn't it also the case where if you are compensating in how you stand or walk to ease the pain in a certain area of your body, then that can cause other issues on the other side of the body because of how you're compensating?*

Dr. Alan Khiger:	Correct. That would be a compensatory mechanical pain just like someone who has a football, basketball, or even baseball injury. If somebody is hit with a baseball thrown at 90 miles an hour, and they get hit in the right knee, while you're going to focus on the right knee, and alleviate the pain on the bad side, you are going to put all this weight distribution on the left knee which will involve all the joints in your body such as your ankle, your hip, your back, your shoulder, and your knee, and that will result over time with chronic compensatory pain on the good side that wasn't really involved from the get-go in the accident.

~	*I would suspect that there is a time frame whether it's one day, or three days, or ten days that you really must get into see a*

Pain in the Wreck

chiropractor after an accident to make sure of the extent of the pain, the hidden damages. How soon should they come in after an accident?

Dr. Alan Khiger: The patient should come immediately after the accident because the patient might be having misdiagnosed concussion symptoms. If they have misdiagnosed concussion symptoms, eventually it could lead in the very serious complications with the brain and the spinal cord. The immediate follow-up, the immediate evaluation should be reserved and exercised immediately after the accident since those injuries are extremely dangerous.

~   *Yes, I can see that definitely. What led you to the field of chiropractic?*

Dr. Alan Khiger: The field of chiropractic basically was led as a result of my own personal injury that I had when I was a kid growing up in Soviet Union. I was climbing up a tree when I was six years old, and

I fell off the tree, but while I was falling off the tree, a twig actually pierced through my knee.

At that point, Soviet Union medicine was not as advance as United States. I wound up going to a hospital and catching an infection which started deteriorating my body over time, and resulting in the condition called osteomyelitis (infection red blood cells that gets produced inside the bone.) That osteomyelitis also started deteriorating my lungs which I had a great formation of pus which is called sepsis. I was in intensive care unit unconscious for 21 days.

Miraculously, I was able to come out of this condition when my grandfather was able to help me with a medicine that he brought overseas because he was in the military service. I was so deteriorated already after that that I had no strength even feed myself because my muscle grade on a possible five out of five was actually zero. The nurses had to actually spoon feed me because of my wasting of the muscles.

Pain in the Wreck

It took me at least four years to recover. This is how long it took me to recover on the injury basically such as that at six years old. You can imagine the recovery process in other patients who are involved in similar situation or similar conditions. Like I said earlier before, these injuries take a very long time to heal.

~ *Your young six-year-old body took that long. Imagine an adult which takes typically much longer. Now, you have your cause and your focus to help others. What made you start your own business as opposed to working for someone else or a clinic?*

Dr. Alan Khiger: When I got into the business, it was basically already a feel of clinical experience that I had gained as a result of managing these conditions. Of course, you don't know everything in medicine just like judges don't know the whole law. To an extent of managing personal injury, I gained a good stable ground on helping out patients recover. Also prepared recommendation which is one of the most important part in this whole arena is we're going to do recommendation for the patient so they can get the proper management, as well as compensation that they deserve for other results of the injuries. Then, I became more confident and more experienced, and that's what led to me operating my own business.

~ *You think about some people that have been involved in a car accident and I would venture to say that one of the first questions is, how long will it take for me to get back to normal? Typically, how long will it take?*

Dr. Alan Khiger: An average, it is minimum 90 days to get back to normal. That, once again, depends on the patient's size, patient's gender, and patient's condition. For example, if the patient has a diagnosis of an inflammatory condition such as arthritis, heart disease, diabetes, of course the healing process is going to take effect a lot longer because the inflammation is the first stage of healing where the body goes through when you get into a car accident.

~ *You mentioned gender. What does gender have to do with how fast that you will get back to your typical quality of life?*

Dr. Alan Khiger: That's a great question but the gender basically is going to impact the female population's the most. Females are prone to deliver babies and go through the process of pregnancy where the whole hormonal process and the functional process gets older for the period of nine months. They deal with some of the conditions that that are similar from the car accident patients which is morning sickness, stiffness, and also an overload on the ligaments which connect bones to bones.

Those ligaments have a tendency to overstretch, and we call it in medicine: laxity.Laxity is one of the bigger deals that it takes a very long time to heal for patients, especially who undergo car accident treatment because of just the geographical position where the ligament is located versus the muscle which is a superficial structure on the body.

Given that, it's going to impact a female who already delivered two or three kids, who already have stressed-out ligaments, who already worked in trying to support the family, and what have you. It's going to exert more pressure on the structures, the neuromuscular skeletal structures such as muscles, bones, disks, nerves, and ligaments. The healing process, once again, takes a lot longer, and the sensitivity to the pain is actually more receptive than a male.

~ *What do you find is the most common obstacle preventing a car accident victim from getting the desired outcome as soon as they want to?*

Dr. Alan Khiger: The compliance is the number one obstacle at getting the desired outcome because compliancy is 90% of the patient's recovery. Just like Woody Allen said, "90% of the success is just showing up." If the patient is not going to be compliant, he is not going to do what needs to be done as opposed to getting better that they're going to fail because you need to have a plan. If you don't have a plan in place, you're bound to fail. There is just no way around it and that's how it works.

~ *What are some of the typical things that you see a patient not following?*

Pain in the Wreck

Dr. Alan Khiger: The patient might get into the moderate improvement without completing the three phrases of healing which I will talk about later. At that point, they feel like, "Okay, I can withdraw from treatment right now because I had gained some moderate results. Quite frankly, the rest will heal on its own. Therefore, I am going to get on with my life, do what I have to do, and stop coming in for treatments."

A lot of times, it's a failed thought process for a lot of patients. They wind up being in a worse situation than they were. Then, they're trying to find a solution for the problem and even giving in to the problem saying, "Look, I admit, it was my fault that I haven't followed the treatment but can you please help me? Can you please help me?"

Of course, the help is always there but the process of restoring what the person has worked for a few weeks coming into the treatment, driving to the treatment, doing the exercises, doing the rehabilitation, stretching, balancing, prospective analysis, and then you're just throwing it away. You could completely throw away the process. At that point, it's completely sad that this patient who could have gotten the complete recovery from their accident or return to pre-accident condition just wind up throwing everything away.

~ *Can you speak to the people that really want to get it done in two months rather than four months, and doing it too fast is not good either?*

Dr. Alan Khiger: Absolutely because once again, they have to bypass the three phases of healing which the first phase is inflammation phase. A great example of that is using ice taking Tylenol or Ibuprofen to suppress the inflammation. This is where the body goes through a reconstructive process. Then, it requires more intensive approach where they have to come in sometimes every day for treatment depending on what phase they are.

Then, once they completed the inflammation phase, intensive care phase, the body gets into the second phase of healing which is called the repair phase. The repair phase, this is when the ligaments, the tendons, the muscles, the disks, and the nerves, they begin to repair. At that point, that stage requires four weeks of commitment for treatment.

Now, once they complete the second phase of healing, then they jump to the last phase of healing which is called the remodeling phase. The remodeling phase is the phase when the nerves, the tendons, the ligaments, the disks, they go into the remodel. It's the same thing as when you have a cut on your finger, you bleed from the cut, the bleeding stops, and then you have a scar for the rest of your life. All of these phases need to take place in order for the body to achieve the absolute required healing to get to the pre-accident status.

~ *It's almost like the concept that you have three hours to cut down a tree, you should spend the first hour sharpening your axe so that you're ready to efficiently cut down the tree. Many people think, "Let's just jump right in and push through these phases," but in reality, your body needs to have that progression so that one phase can build off of the other.*

Dr. Alan Khiger: Yes, correct. Unfortunately, this is how the mechanism physiologically is designed and there is nothing that we can do about it. Just like you have a gravitational force on earth, you have a zero gravitational force on the moon.

~   *What do you find is the biggest misconceptions or pitfalls that people might not be aware of before they start their treatment that they need to be, about what to expect?*

Dr. Alan Khiger: They have to understand that this is a very destructive process in terms of what it could do on the financial burden for the patient. For example, if somebody has a family, if it's a single mom and if she is not going to take advantage of the treatment for the injury that's associated with a car accident, that's going to create an economic hardship for the mom to provide for the family because think about it, if she's going to get to a point where she's not going to be able to go back to work and doing the duties that she's got to do at work, what's going to happen then to the family that she's got to feed to the kids, they got to be fed, and buying clothes, get them to school, give them lunch money, etc. if she's unwilling to perform the duties at her job.

That is basically what's at stake on these injuries. Also, the emotional component when patients are winding up with no car and they're thinking, "What's going to happen next? I don't think I am going to recover from this. This is something I never felt before." All of these factors could come in as a shock to someone who has all these different situations that they're involved in. That's an emotional component that's pretty much got to be dealt with primarily when someone is going through this painful process.

~ *It sounds like there's some very tangible literal things that you prepare the patients for. One of them is what you just touched on which is the emotional aspect of how they should be preparing. Can you speak about both the physical and the emotional preparations that let the patient know, "You're going to experience this, and it's okay, and it's normal"?*

Dr. Alan Khiger

Dr. Alan Khiger: Yeah, because everybody is going to have some

characteristics of recovery that's resonating with other patients who are

coming in for treatment. One of the things that we prepare the patient

for the worse outcome, we sit down with the patient and pretty much

from day one, we give the patient an estimate of how long the treatment

will take place, what to expect during the treatment, what type of home

therapies that they can go through to prepare the healing process, and

how long they need to be staying out of work for, providing the

communication for the work depending on what type of duties it

requires for them to perform for the employer.

Also, we pretty much get the family involved doing the

intervention if someone has a loved one and they have dependency. We

take all measures necessary to have this patient be comfortable and

ready to deal with those injuries. Sometimes, if we have pediatric

patients and they have been exposed to this horror, obviously, we'll

refer them to a psychological evaluation or psychiatric evaluation. Then,

they co-treat with the psychological or psychiatric professional together so they can achieve the best healing process for their emotional and psychological condition.

~ *In that example, it sounds like there are some cases requiring more than one clinician to get involved. You mentioned the psychological assessment. What other types of professionals would you bring in to help with their treatment protocol?*

Dr. Alan Khiger: We also bring in the orthopedic professionals. We also bring in the medical doctor professionals. We also bring in the pain management professionals who are working together with us to co-treat those conditions because, like I said, a lot of times, these injuries have a different classification. If you have broken bones involved, or lacerations, or punctured lung, or punctured kidney, or broken bone, of course, that will require a more intellectual approach of getting those professionals who I just mentioned to manage those conditions. That, of course, will require more than 90 days for the patient to get better if warranted.

Dr. Alan Khiger

~   *I think that a lot of people have a misconception that if I go to*

a chiropractor that's turning my back on the medical community and

that you're describing that you embrace working all of the

communities together from the orthopedic, to the medical, to the

psychological, and that's a very healthy approach. I am sure that

patients appreciate that.

Dr. Alan Khiger: Yes, they do because we found out throughout

the clinical experience that the patients would be a lot more receptive to

other forms of treatment which are more integrative. That's what we

implement in our practice to give the patient more of an option to get

better and feel comfortable with the treatment, with what we provide.

~   *Can you think of an example of an injury that was unique, and*

you helped them work through that, and then maybe another example

of what a more common accident victim would be experiencing, and

some of the things that they can expect?

Pain in the Wreck

Dr. Alan Khiger: Yes. We had a patient who was a family of four, and she was involved in an accident where she wound up actually with a broken talus, (which is a bone in the foot), and also there was a kidney laceration which resulted for a broken rib bone puncturing the organ. We were managing this patient for spinal condition disorders such as irritation of the nervous system, leakage in the disk, also strain of the ligaments, sprain of the muscles. That patient took at least two years to heal because of so much going on with her. We were, of course, managing her for the conditions that I just mentioned earlier before.

Then, we had to refer her out to the psychologist after we were finished with the chiropractic here, and we had to refer her to the follow-up for the orthopedic professionals who had manage her for the fractured foot bone. Also, she was seeing an internist for the laceration of the kidney. All in all, it took, like I said earlier, for the patient to get stable at least a year and still continued treatment for two years for the broken talus, and the lacerated kidney.

Dr. Alan Khiger

Another case study that we had that was a construction worker who basically had a rare condition in the spine. He had anomaly of his bones in the lower back. He was basically misdiagnosed by prior physicians on this anomaly which is called Facet Tropism. Facet Tropism is pretty much irregular aligning of your spine that automatically limits your range of motion. You're already born with a chronic low back condition for the rest of your life. Can you imagine if somebody gets into a car accident, how that person will feel?

This was a healthy, young fellow in his late 20s who was muscular. He was extremely happy of the procedure or model of treatment that we allocated for him and the rehab that actually was a very good fit for his particular type of condition that helped him get back to normal. He wound up going back to work and doing all the complicated construction work, going on the roof, gathering all the sheetrock that is extremely heavy. He was very pleased, and he was happy, and still able to do physical labor coming out of a very serious injury like I just mentioned earlier before.

Pain in the Wreck

We pride ourselves in managing those conditions and referring patients to the appropriate medical doctors to help us get the maximum improvement on the patient.

~ ***Are you ever asked by people from the insurance companies, of pre-existing conditions? Is there any way to prove that?***

Dr. Alan Khiger: Yeah, that's a very good question, because a lot of times, patients might have a pre-existing condition but once again, once you have a pre-existing condition and you get into an accident, that's going to exacerbate that condition. We ask the patient prior to the treatment what was his pain like before he was involved in an accident. We question the frequency, intensity, and duration of his pain. Then, we question the intensity, duration, and frequency of his pain after the accident, following up with the imaging such as x-rays and MRI.

Then, we sit down with the patient and pretty much go over the imaging of the MRI and x-ray, and show this patient how his injury prior to that was impacted by the accident, and where he's at right now, and what type of injury that he has now as a result of the old injury he had prior to that. This is one of the ways that we use to separate the old injury from the new injury.

~ *That's really important. You were mentioning imaging and x-rays. I am sure that you work very closely with the insurance companies because they're the ones that are approving payments for the treatment. Can you speak to how that is taken care of with the insurance companies and is there anything to keep in mind such as if you have too many tests done at the hospital that might not leave funds for the chiropractic?*

Dr. Alan Khiger: Yeah. A lot of times, if the patient has suffered a serious injury and he called the ambulance on the scene to transport the patient into the hospital, the hospital might perform certain diagnostic imaging such as CT scans which are going to be extremely expensive. They range between $8,000 to $10,000.

Pain in the Wreck

If you have only $10,000 left on the medical side for your car accident injuries; which is a state law in Florida. Whether you're at fault, whether you caused the accident or whether you are a victim of someone who caused the accident, you have $10,000 that is set for your medical expenses. If you're going to go to the hospital after the ambulance transports you at the scene, and the hospital decides that it was necessary for them to do the CT scan, and the CT scan came out negative, then the patient is going to be in the hole at $9000, and none of his other injuries are going to be addressed.

At that point, the patient is pretty much left with two options. He could either use an attorney lien that will protect him and have the patient at fault reimburse him for other further expenses, or they could use the medical health insurance to continue with treatment. This is pretty much one of the things that sometimes becomes problematic for our patients because the CT scan was maybe necessary by the hospital and it didn't demonstrate the injury that the hospital thought it was going to demonstrate. Then, it's a huge burden on the patient and causes lots of big problems.

Dr. Alan Khiger

~   Is there a tip or two that a patient should keep in mind when thinking about dealing with the insurance companies? I am sure that a lot of accident victims consider using an attorney or not using an attorney? Is this test going to cost me money that I cannot get reimbursed?

Dr. Alan Khiger: That's a very good question because the first time a patient gets into a car accident; they're going to call the insurance to file a claim. Once they filed a claim, the insurance company is going to ask the patient, "Are you hurt?" The patient can say, "Yes, I am hurt." The insurance company might take this recorded statement from the patient.

Then, the patient might get another phone call from another insurance company or from the party that was involved in the accident and they can say, "Look, we know you're hurt. We can send you a check for $2,000. All you have to do is just sign it, and we'll take care of your medical expenses." Of course, the $2,000 is not nearly enough to someone who is suffering from this long-term whiplash injury condition.

Pain in the Wreck

The best thing is to basically get advice from an attorney. Attorneys will provide free consultation for the most part for anybody who is in a car accident. At least, there will be advice of their rights of how to respond to the insurance company. Of course, they're the ones who are going to be making that decision.

~ I think that that's very important and so many things are happening immediately upon the accident. They're worried, they're scared, they're disoriented, what would your best piece of advice be to the car accident victim who is now the ... Immediately once that happens, what's the best piece of advice to take that next step? Who is the first call?

Dr. Alan Khiger: The first set of action is basically get clearance on the injury. The clearance on the injury is going to come from us. That's what we're going to provide. We're going to provide a comprehensive orthopedic neurological examination which will pretty much encompass and entail if the patient was indeed hurt as a result of the accident along with the diagnostic imaging. We would then sit down and show the patient that there has been an alteration in the bones in their spine, there has been alteration in the ligament. There has been a malfunction in the muscles. There has been loss of sensation on their skin due to the nerve insufficiency or impingement.

We are going to be looking at all of those factors in detail and provide the patient then a hypothetical report where then, the patient then pretty much makes his decision whether they want to follow a treatment or not. Of course, the second step would be providing them with the advice to seek an attorney for the injuries.

~ *Yeah, that's super important. What's another important thing that the car accident victim should think about if they're worried that chiropractic care may not work for them or might not apply to their situation?*

Dr. Alan Khiger: If they have neuromuscular skeletal complications, then they should be getting better after they complete the inflammation phase (which is the first phase in healing). If they don't get better after they complete the intensive phase of healing, obviously, this patient needs to be referred out, but the patient always is going to need some type of medical care after they get into accident.

Because just think about this one, you have a 5,000-pound cars that runs into an average person who is 180 pounds. That person is going to have some reaction to this impact. It doesn't matter because you just can't say that you're not hurt after a 5,000-pound car runs into your body. It's impossible. It's like saying somebody could jump above an eight-story building. Can they do it? If they have some super hero traits, and how often is that? Maybe you could say somebody say that they are Superman and they have a 1% heroic trait, they don't feel anything, then maybe I could agree with that but 99.9%, that's not the case. You will have an irritation into the nervous system.

Just like if somebody ambushes your body or you're a football player, you get run over by a 250-pound linebacker, you are going to have the irritation of your nervous system. Just like you are going partying, drinking, and then you have to wake up two hours later to go to work, your body is going to be irritated. You're going to be irritated. You're going to have irritated responses to someone who is trying to communicate with you and that's essentially what is going on when you get into this motor vehicle trauma.

~ *What are some of the fears that people commonly have when working with a chiropractor?*

Dr. Alan Khiger: The first common fear that they have is, "The treatment is not going to work on me because I am so injured, I am so messed up, I am going to give up. I am going to prepare to live with pain for the rest of my life." That's the number one fear.

The second fear is, "It's going to cost me a lot of money. I am going to be winding up with a lot of medical bills. It's going to be devastating for my family. We're always going to be owing money for these medical bills." The third one is actually, "I'm not going to be able to get through this because the hours are not feasible for me because I am working until 6:00 or 7:00 in the evening. I may not be able to come in." A conflicting schedule.

All of these fear factors are taken into consideration in our facility. We explain to patients pretty much what the customary bill of the treatment would be once they start treatment with us. We explain to the patient what percentage of improvement they expect to gain in the first three weeks, and then the next four weeks, and the next following weeks. With the projected prognosis, we reexamine the patient after all of those trimesters, the system that we have.

Pretty much, we tell the patient, "We encourage you for sticking to this treatment plan because it was explained to you earlier before that you're going to gain X amount of percentage to get better. Therefore, you did it. Now, you actually did well as you did before. Do you currently have any other things that you're worrying about in life that perhaps would not have you be committed to treatment?"

We call them out on the first day. Then, we also ask them, "On a scale of zero to ten, how committed are you to care? If we don't get a solid ten, if we get an eight, we'll say, "What are some of the things that you might not be a ten?" They'll pretty much admit to having a conflicted schedule, not being able to come in four times a week versus three times a week. We're trying to get all the possible objections out there to come up with a comprehensive solution for the patient's problem because first and foremost, we are problem solvers at the Amazing Spine Care.

~ *I think that a lot of people would also have a fear that chiropractic treatment may cause more damage because they're already hurt from the accident?*

Dr. Alan Khiger: Basically, we can have different types of chiropractic approaches. We could use hands-on approach which will be manipulation via hand or we could use a more noninvasive approach such as Activator which is using an instrument which is a lot lighter on the body versus chiropractic treatment. That's what we do primarily with younger adult population and geriatric population which are receptive to that type of treatment. Also, we tend to ask in the beginning what are some of the negative things that they have heard about chiropractic that they haven't heard before. Pretty much, we will present the solution for the best chiropractic approach for this patient.

~ *You mentioned nervous system. I think that that's something that a lot of people do not associate with chiropractic care because it's not the bones, it's not the muscles. How does the nervous system get impacted negatively from this car accident?*

Dr. Alan Khiger: The nervous system is pretty much a wire that carries communication in our body to the brain. Without the nervous system, we would not even be alive or functional because first, when we are a fetus, the fetus is actually a notochord remnant of our nervous system. It looks like a bean. Then, that bean pretty much grows in the other structures such as bones, disks, ligaments, tendons, muscle which is called development. During this development, our nervous system is the key player into those milestones that we go through.

33

When you have an impact on the spine, the nerves that run pretty much parallel and they go into the legs, they're located on the back, they go in to the arms, they're located in the neck, if the patient had some impact by the car, whether it's coming from the side in a T-bone collision or coming from the back in a rear-end collision, it's going to affect each never specifically.

For example, the injuries that we found out in our experience which resulted in a T-bone collision were a lot more hurtful to the patient because of the geographical location of these nerves which is called the plexus. The plexus irritation feels a lot longer than, for example, someone might get in the back. We question the mechanism of the injury first to take a procedural care plan for this patient. Then, we explain why the irritation of the nerves, in retrospect to the position, how the body was damaged from is going to heal.

~ *It's amazing how many things are connected in the body, and then how one impactful accident can throw off so many systems. What do you do about patients that are going to face constant chronic pain*

because of the accident? As much as you can help them with the pain

they're still going to deal with it, what do you do to give them hope

that it can be managed?

Dr. Alan Khiger: When we put them on the extensive care plan, we

let them know that even after they finish their treatment, they have to

self-manage their condition. Insurance companies also require doctors

these days to have the patients educated on using the proper exercises

for keeping their spinal hygiene. Those exercises pretty much worked

through and performed by the patient on a per visit basis. The patient

has a whole lot of information to take home after they finish their

treatment with us.

The patient is advised from the get-go that it's not the injuries

and the pain itself they're going to have to go through while they're

undergoing treatment, it's basically what's going to happen to them

after they finish their treatment. That's the most important part because

if they don't follow up with the particular exercise protocol, if they don't follow up with a particular spinal hygiene protocol, those injuries will come back. These patients will suffer exactly the same type of injuries as they had from day one when they got into this accident.

If they want to be healthy, if they want to match the gains that they got as a result of the accident, they have to be committed to following the protocol of those exercises on a daily basis just like brushing their teeth. If they don't brush their teeth every day, what's going to happen to the patient's teeth? They're pretty much aware that the teeth are going to rot, they're going to turn to a different color. The same analogy applies to the spine. Spine is the same type of bone of a tooth. It's all bone and tissue. Once you have a bone and tissue, you have to sustain a certain type of hygiene for that bone to have somewhat of a manageable lifestyle after they complete their treatment.

~ *Have you had patients where they finish your treatment protocol, and their accident injuries were managed and treated well, and then they also noticed that some previous injuries or previous conditions they had have also been fixed through your treatment protocol, and they never would have thought to come in to see you had it not been for the accident?*

Dr. Alan Khiger: Yes. We had a patient who basically was in a second accident. He was complaining of a neck, mid back, lower back, and shoulder pain. While undergoing treatment, he started having severe stomach pain. We basically referred the patient out to our primary care medical doctor who manages patients who have a vehicle trauma. The medical doctor had told them that, "You actually need to do some blood work and take care of this problem in your stomach, whatever condition that you're describing to us."

The patient did not listen. Towards the end of the treatment, he wound up actually having such a severe stomach pain that he was hospitalized, and he wind up undergoing a surgery for the gallbladder and also wind up with a $50,000 bill on top of it. Then, the patient wound up coming back to us, and admitting to the fact that he wasn't the patient who was compliant to listen to what was going on.

Dr. Alan Khiger

Once again, it goes back to what we're talking about earlier, that the patients have to be compliant not just on the injuries that they're coming to see us for, but also on other injuries that they have coming from different parts of their bodies.

After all, we are doctors who are dealing with patients who have all types of different disorders and those patients need to be managed for these conditions because it can, again, become aggravated and it can play a big role in reinjuring the patient again emotionally and physically.

~   *You mentioned the symbiotic synergy relationship between the medical community and bringing in extra practitioners. Do you also have the same connection with the doctors who are prescribing medication and you may also prescribe additional vitamins or things like that to help the healing process?*

Dr. Alan Khiger: Yes, we do. We recommend to patients nutritional vitamins for healing such as vitamin C which works great for healing the tissues, also Vitamin B. Also, we recommend magnesium for the muscle spasms. In the primary intensive care, we refer the patient out for the prescription medication that the patient might need. Then, of course, the medical doctor makes a decision of what type of prescriptions that they want to put the patient on, and being that we have a crisis with the overprescribed medication these days, we'll make sure that the patient has been carefully prescribed the type of medication that would be comfortable for his tolerance while he's undergoing treatment.

~   *Are there ever any protocols that you would see that you would make a recommendation on regarding medication where they may form a drug dependency where maybe the best course of action would be some vitamins or some supplements?*

Dr. Alan Khiger: We always recommend but we cannot prescribe since we don't have the license. We can only advise to the patient to speak to the medical doctor who has the discretion to adjust medication or take them off the medication if necessary.

~   Yes, that's excellent, are there are some things that you would make recommendations on regarding the treatment protocol as it relates to vitamins, supplements, and that could help recovery along. What about something as simple as extra sleep, extra water, things like that that they can be doing at home that would help recovery?

Dr. Alan Khiger: Yeah, absolutely. Once the patient has gone through a certain amount of treatment, days or weeks, in our clinic, then they found themselves sleeping a lot better. They also find themselves that they're able to be more well rested. That's, of course, due to the impact on the nervous system.

Now, another thing that we highly recommend is basically hydration or water which would then rehydrate the disks that are damaged in the spine because once you have an injury to those disks and we refer them out for an imaging of MRI, then if the MRI comes in positive for disk herniation, or disk bulge, what have you, then we're going to recommend the patient drinking as much water as possible.

Pain in the Wreck

Of course, we provide the bottles of water in our clinic when the patient comes in to see us and we let them know the importance of water, how it is imperative that it gets into those disks. They need to be hydrated to maintain the pressure on the nerves that are currently impinged or compressed by the bone above during an accident.

~ *I think just water is such a simple thing to overlook. The way you just described that with keeping the pressure to keep things working the right way and to keep the disk from being too brittle, or the fluid in there, the water impact so much of that.*

Do you find that some people fight you on that?

Dr. Alan Khiger: There's going to be all different types of patients who have all different types of preferences. Of course, you're going to have patients who are coffee drinkers and coffee is going to impact the pituitary gland for more demand of fluids because it's going to also increase the kidney into urinating more often because it's a diuretic.

Then, the patient is going to wind up losing more fluids than they're actually putting into their body. With the coffee drinkers, it becomes a little more problematic because they're going to dehydrate all the necessary fluids and water for the tendons and ligaments which I mentioned earlier before who have that unique geographic location in the body and the oxygen that's necessary for those ligaments and tendons are very difficult to get into to achieve the desired healing process for the patient.

Therefore, we're trying to explain to the patient the consequences of having too much caffeine in their system. If the patient, for example, says, "Look, I have preference. I just don't like the water taste." Of course, we're going to say, "That's fine. Then, you can choose the fluids of your preference. For example, you can have an iced tea but you have to make sure that you don't have the other factors such as sodium or sugar which can potentially lead to other consequences because if you're going to have sodium, for example, in the liquid that you are consuming, you're going to spike up your blood pressure."

That's not going to sit well with somebody who is chronic hypertensive patient.

Also, if you have someone who is overweight or obese, the sugary liquid substances are going to retain that sugar and overnight turn into fat where the patients are going to be getting more weight, and that would slow down the healing process if they're undergoing all the three phases of healing. These are the factors that have to be set in place and explained to the patient who has some misunderstanding and misconceptions of how the water intake can benefit them or harm them.

~   *You mentioned previously about sleep. Do you recommend more sleep during the recovery process? Is there a certain sleep posture that they need to be thinking about?*

Dr. Alan Khiger: Yes, absolutely. The posture is always a big factor especially with someone who has an abnormal posture from the get-go. That's one of the primary diagnosis that we use in our recommendations for the patient's protocol. Also, that is a further workup that we do with the patient once they begin their rehab therapeutic activity protocol. That's definitely going to be a factor for the patient who is not able to have a comfortable sleep cycle. We work on the experience of the patient using, for example, towels in between their legs once they go to sleep so they can have that stress taken over on their spine.

We also recommend having the proper mattress that they could sleep on. For example, if the patient says, "My mattress is too soft." If your mattress is too soft, that is not going to provide the adequate support for the bones and the muscles. Therefore, the patient is going to wind themselves hurting more in the mornings because there was no stability and support. For example, if the patient is going to have a mattress that is so rough, that's going to hurt the patient's bones, and they're going to wind up being hurt as well.

There has to be a balance, yin yang in between the mattress, also the adequate sleeping position for the patient such as using the pillows in between the legs, and also lean on the side and try to have a proper alignment for the spine to heal properly.

~ *Can you give us final thoughts on what an accident victim would need to keep in mind regarding seeking the proper care? Then, what is the best way for someone that's been involved in an accident to learn more about your practice? Is the best way a website or just to come visit your practice?*

Dr. Alan Khiger: The best way is basically get at first evaluation with us. Other methods would be checking out our website. I speak three languages. I speak Russian, Spanish, and English. We also go with these injuries in all three different languages trying to explain it to the public. This way, there's no barrier as to the availability and what can we do.

Also, the long hours, the after-hours to accommodate the scheduling for the clinic. That's what we provide for the public so they can pretty much come on after work, and get their treatment and the

therapies to accommodate the injuries.

Learn More:

BUSINESS: Amazing Spine Care

WEBSITE: www.AmazingSpineCare.com

EMAIL: amazingspinecare@gmail.com

PHONE: (904) 701-3916

Appendix | Additional Resources

Figure 1.8. This is an illustration of part of the cervical spine (black portion of inset). Part is cut in half for better viewing. This illustrates all of the lesions that have been reported to occur in whiplash trauma. With permission from Whiplash! A Patient's Guide to Recovery. San Diego, (c) Spine Research Institute of San Diego, 1999.

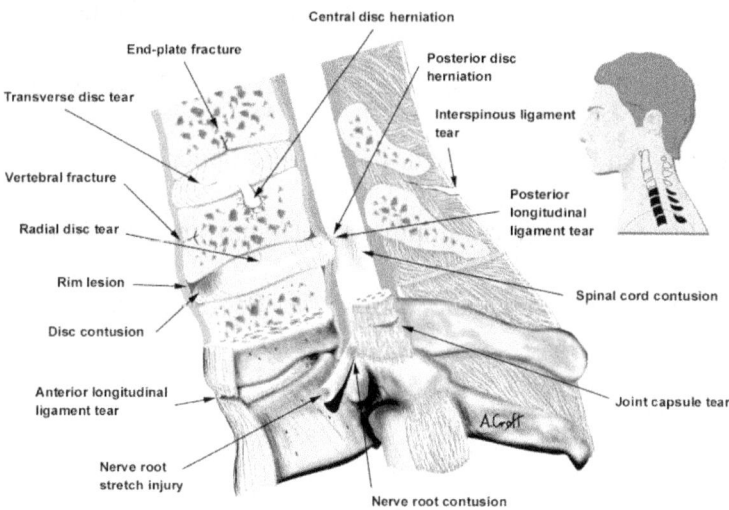

One of the interesting recent findings was that the two most common segments to be affected in an Australian CAD fluoroscopic anesthetic block study were C2-3 and C5-6, with a much greater occurrence on the right than on the left (1333). Note that this is an Australian study and they, like their British cousins, drive on the wrong side of the car. As seen during the s-shaped curve, the upper and lower segments are most affected.

This is also consistent with the PMHS tests.

The most recent literature points also strongly toward the facet joint as a major contributor to neck pain. Kaneoka et al. (1273) referred to the pinching that can be seen to occur in this joint under dynamic crash testing as facet synovial fold impingement syndrome. Siegmund et al. (1495) have offered evidence in quasi-static PMHH tests for the possibility of facet joint capsular ligament injury in whiplash.

Experimental neurophysiological support is offered by Thunberg et al. (1442). They demonstrated that, in cats, the fusimotor-muscle spindle system is subject to a positive feedback error initiated by either (in the context of this study) chemosensory excitation of receptors in the facet joints or mechanoreceptor activity. We are drawn back to the facet joint itself as a major source of neck pain, with muscle stiffness as a likely concomitant factor.

Neck stiffness. Stiffness may be the result of protective muscle spasm secondary to most injuries of the neck. Chronic stiffness indicates myofascial fibrosis or contraction, ligamentous contraction (particularly of joint capsules), disc degeneration, or secondary osteoarthritic change.

Shoulder pain. This can be either from direct injury to the shoulder, such as from a shoulder harness, or impact with the car's interior, or from referred pain from soft tissues of the neck or a disc lesion. Other causes of shoulder pain, such as impingement syndrome, thoracic outlet syndrome (TOS) (1522), and rotator cuff inflammation, may develop secondary to CAD trauma, either as a result of muscular disuse or paresis of muscles or muscle groups. Imbalance between agonist and antagonist muscles can precipitate shoulder disorders or convert subclinical
conditions to clinical conditions. In one study, 53% of the patients were found to have a periarticular shoulder disorder (131).

Dr. Alan Khiger

In a recent study of 476 CAD injury subjects the incidence of impingement-type pain was found to be 9% (1567). Notably, all of the shoulder complaints were delayed in onset. About 12.3% of cases with shoulder pain not diagnosed as impingement syndrome were thought to be the

result of referred pain. Most had abnormal scapulohumeral rhythm motion. Scapulohumeral motion is known to be a composite of glenohumeral and scapulothoracic motion. The trapezius is believed to play a role in abnormalities in this motion in CAD patients.

In an uncontrolled, poorly described report, a group of surgeons reported their success using a combination of arthroscopic shoulder stabilization surgery and brachial plexus neuroloysis (1569). These surgical procedures were not described in detail and the authors methods of patient

selection, inclusion/exclusion criteria, statistical analysis, and outcome assessment were not provided, other than the assessment of two-point discrimination.

Pain in the Wreck

Observing the replay of our high speed video coverage of human subject crash tests, I made saw an interesting phenomenon. A male subject had been warned not to grip the steering wheel. For some reason, even after such exhortations, subjects very often do grip the wheel. At impact, the car is essentially thrust forward beneath the subject. This grip results in a violent stretching of the upper extremity and a pulling of the glenohumeral joint. It also acts to accentuate the extension of the neck. It seems likely that under such circumstances, direct shoulder injuries might occur.

Headaches. These are the result of either injury to the upper cervical spine, or reflex or protective muscle spasm in the neck. Trauma can also play an important role in converting postural faults into clinical headaches (105). Headaches are also attributed to TMJ dysfunction and, rarely,
the Barré-Liéou syndrome. Magnússon et al. (1200) reported that headaches with both a frontal and occipital component responded best to surgical release in cases of occipital neuralgia. Rather than suggesting surgery as a treatment for these patients, I present this for its differential

diagnostic value.

Interscapular pain: This pain is caused either by direct injury to paraspinal muscles or, more commonly, as a result of referred (scleratogenous) pain from the neck. It also may be seen with disc lesions. In the chronic stage, one of the most common causes of this type of pain is myofascial pain disorder (MPD), which is chiefly a secondary effect.

Back pain. Croft and Foreman (315) found low back pain (LBP) in 57% of their CAD cases (71% in broadside collisions). Most recently we've confirmed this relationship (1240). Braaf and Rosner (316) found LBP in 42% of their cases. Hohl (240) found LBP in 35% of his cases. Twenty-five percent of the patients in Hildingsson and Toolanen's study (121) had low back pain. In a recent study of chiropractic therapy in CAD patients, it was found that patients with low back pain generally required more treatment than those with neck pain alone (349). In a prospective study, Gargan and Bannister (456) reported 32% of their group as having LBP and an additional 10% developed LBP as a late manifestation. This same percentage (32%) was found by Bring and Westman (450). Magnússon (131) reported an incidence of 48% with LBP.

In their recent follow-up of 35 patients followed for an average of 10.8 years, Watkinson et al. (249) found that initially, 24% of the group complained of LBP. Of these, 5% resolved later. However, after a 10.8 year mean follow-up, 34% complained of low back pain. It probably represents chronic postural adaptations to pain that, in most cases, developed later. Squires et al. (1201) followed previously studied patients (242,249) and reported a prevalence of back pain in half of this group after 15 years. More recently 40.5% of Brison et al. (1329) group of rear impacted subjects had low back pain at 24 month follow-up. And Jakobsson et al. (1443) found thoracic and lumbar spine injuries second only to cervical injuries in rear impact crashes. In a recent study it was found that of those with neck pain following CAD, 43% of females and 31% of males also had back pain--a statistic that is found frequently in this literature (1368).

The exact mechanism of low back injury in rear impact collisions, although not entirely clear, is probably multifactorial. Factors affecting the incidence, nature, and severity of low back injury in automobile crashes include the following: (1) position of the occupant in vehicle, (2) the use or non-use of seat belts and shoulder harness, (3) deployment of airbag system, (which are designed to deploy only with frontal impacts, but may deploy in more severe secondary collisions), (4) type of restraint system (i.e., conventional restraints vs. restraints with pretensioners), (5) stiffness of the seat back, (6) inclination of the seat back, (7) properties of the seat back padding, (8) degree of ramping, (9) vector and severity of the collision, (10) second collisions inside or outside the occupant's vehicle, (11) snugness of the restraint system, (12) positioning of the restraint system on the occupant, (13) positioning of the restraint system anchors within the vehicle, (14) physical makeup of the occupant, including stature, build, age, and level of fitness, and (15) preparedness for the collision.

Frontal impacts are the most frequent type of crash and are also responsible for the most severe injuries. However, controlling for the severity of the crash (i.e., the actual amount of force involved), injuries

are much more frequent in rear impact collisions. One of the prime

reasons for this is that drivers who hit other cars are typically aware of

the impending collision in time to brace for the impact. Steering wheels,

brake pedals, and floorboards, in combination with the ride down of

vehicle crush, provide adequate additional support to prevent many

injuries.

In side impacts, the occupants of most production car seats are offered

little protection to lateral acceleration forces by either seat back or

restraint system. This probably explains why Dr. Foreman and I found

such a high incidence of low back pain following this type of collision.

[Incidentally, it was later Dr. Freeman and I who confirmed this

relationship (1240).] The initial response to broadside impact is lateral

flexion toward the striking vehicle, with compression of spinal

structures on the concave side and stretching of myofascial and other

structures on the convex side. The lap belt will serve as an anchor for

the pelvis thus preventing serious injury. It may, however, intensify

bending moments in the lumbosacral or thoracolumbar spine, thus increasing the likelihood of soft tissue injury. Intervertebral disc injuries, as well as ligamentous and muscular injuries, are common.

Broadside collisions should be analyzed carefully. Forces incurred by striking and struck vehicles are not commonly perfectly perpendicular. For example, if a broadside collision occurs between two cars in an intersection, and both are traveling at 20 mph, the actual resulting vectors of deceleration for the occupants will be oblique to the direction they are traveling in: in the case of the car that is struck on the driver's side, the occupant will decelerate in a vector that is forward and toward the striking car; in the case of the striking car, the occupant will decelerate forward and opposite to the direction the other car. Such oblique collisions are particularly difficult to describe both kinetically and kinematically. However, it is clear from studies conducted by Viano (206) that oblique rear impact collisions hold much greater potential for injury than the pure rear impact variety. This is also true for other vectors of collision.

Pain in the Wreck

Occupants wearing only a lap belt are more vulnerable to lumbar injury than those wearing a three-point system as a result of the tendency to rebound forward immediately after loading the seat back in the acceleration stage of a rear impact collision. Shoulder straps will mitigate some of the inertia of the decelerating trunk. We found that seat belt use did not contribute to chronicity of low back pain (1240). Several studies have demonstrated the potential to ramp up the seat back after rear impact collision. This tendency is even greater in out-of-position occupants (205).

The initial effect of ramping will be abrupt axial stretch of the lumbar spine with compression of the cervical spine. This stretch will still be felt if the pelvis is firmly anchored by the lap belt and ramping is thus prevented. Many occupants slouch and/or lean forward in their car seats. In either case, the first area of the body to be accelerated by the seat back will be the pelvis. This bending moment will effectively flex the lumbosacral spine until the thorax comes into full contact with the seat back. As the seat back is loaded with elastic energy from the inertia of the occupant, it will extend backward in proportion to these forces--a movement that can exceed 30 degrees. At this time significant slack can develop in the restraint belts (particularly the shoulder belt) and the excess webbing may not be spooled back into the retractors (80). Then, as the head and torso decelerate in the forward direction, carried along by a combination of their own inertia and the released elastic energy from the seat back, this slack is overcome suddenly, resulting in acute peaks in deceleration forces and subjecting the lumbar spine to its second flexion injury, this time in combination with the shear force provided by the restraining lap belt. In this case the inertia of the pelvis and lower extremities may be relatively unrestrained and can carry the lower half of the body against the belt. If the occupant is fully braced against the brake or floorboards, this effect will be significantly minimized.

Recently a cadaver was instrumented with rosette strain gauges applied on the lateral and anterior surfaces of T12, L2, and L4 and subjected to rear impacts of 5g and 8g (1533). The authors reported that the forces generated during simulated whiplash collision were of insufficient magnitude to cause bony injuries, but they may be sufficient to cause soft-tissue injuries. Cassidy et al. (1548) reported that "low back pain is a common traffic injury with a prolonged recovery. Its incidence and prognosis are affected by multiple factors, including the type of compensation system. Our study suggests that biopsychosocial factors are important in determining prognosis." "Suggested," in this case, is an accurate term, as opposed to "demonstrated." The study can be criticized in a number of ways.

Some of the preceding potential factors for lumbar injury are illustrated in Figure 1.9.

Figure 2.8. The Principal direction of force (PDOF) of colliding vehicles is indicated by arrows. Occupant motions will follow these lines. This is an oversimplification of the PDOF, however. As Brach and Brach note (recommended reading 4), without experience and knowledge in impulse mechanics, the PDOF can be difficult to determine accurately.

PICTURE

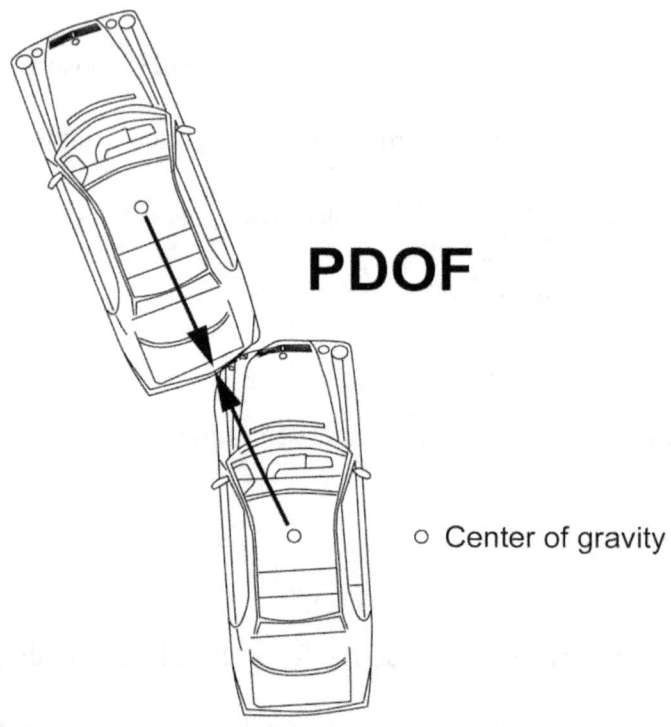

PDOF

○ Center of gravity

PICTURE 8261Figure 2.16. In the case of offset rear impact, the target

vehicle, depending on crash speed and road condition, may rotate

around its own

center of gravity. The occupant will experience both linear and

rotational acceleration, A. Rotation of the vehicle to the left would

produce the same neck loads as would a non-offset rear impact vector

crash in which the occupant's head was rotated to the right, B.

(Adapted from reference 1402.)

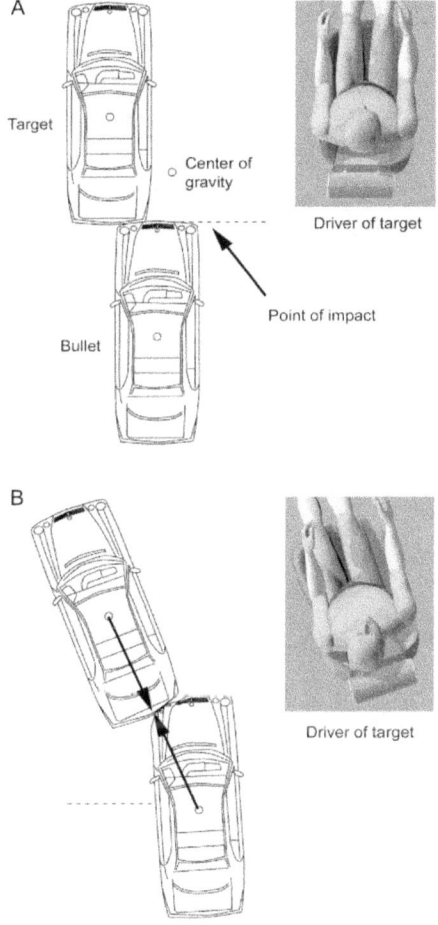

Figure 2.17. In the case of oblique rear impact collisions, a combination of linear and rotational acceleration and asymmetric facet loading will nearly always occur, A and B.

(Adapted from reference 1402.) PICTURE 83

Dr. Alan Khiger

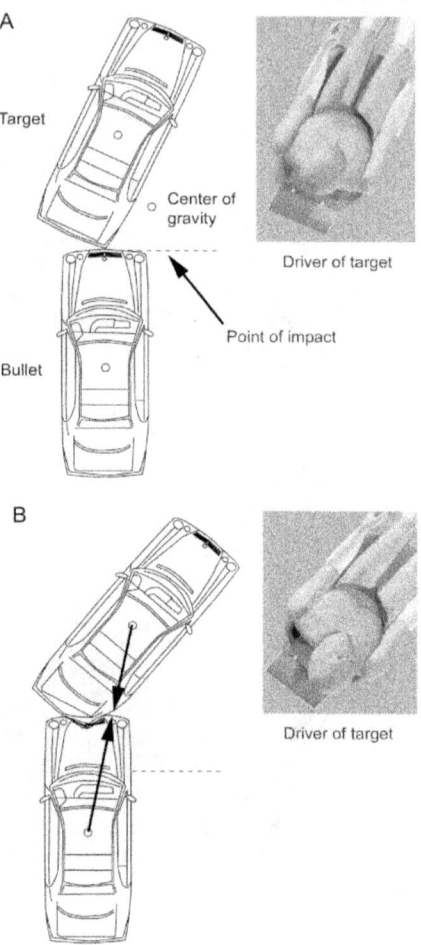

A

Target

Center of gravity

Driver of target

Point of impact

Bullet

B

Driver of target

- In 1964, the *Journal of Bone and Joint Surgery (American)* published a study where the author followed 145 whiplash-injured patients for more than two years. The author reported that after a minimum of two years, between 45% to 83% of the injured patients continued to suffer from pain.*

- The author's study initially included 266 injured patients, but at the follow-up assessment (more than 2 years later) only 145 were evaluated (121 of the original group were not evaluated at the two plus year follow-up). Of the 145 followed patients, 83% were still suffering pain symptoms. The author noted that if he assumed that   100% of the 121 subjects who were not evaluated were completely symptom free, then the incidence of chronic pain in the entire initial   266 patient set fell to 43%.

- In 1989, the journal *Neuro-Orthopedics* published a 12.5-year (mean duration) study on whiplash-injured patients. The authors reported that 62% continued to suffer from significant pain symptoms attributed to the motor vehicle collision 12.5 years later.

- In 2000, the *Journal of Clinical Epidemiology* published a 7-year study on whiplash-injured patients. The authors reported that 39.6% continued to suffer from neck-shoulder pain 7 years after injury. This 39.6% chronic pain rate was three times greater than the pain noted in the matched control populations.

- In 2005, the journal *Injury* published a 7.5 year prospective study on whiplash-injured patients. The authors reported that 21% of these patients continued to suffer from clinically relevant pain 7.5 years after injury. An additional 48% continued to suffer from nuisance pain at the 7.5-year analysis.

- In 1990, the *Journal of Bone and Joint Surgery (British)* published a 10.8 year study on whiplash-injured patients. The authors reported that 40% of these patients continued to suffer from clinically significant pain 10.8 years after injury. An additional 40% continued to suffer from nuisance pain at the 10.8-year analysis.

- In 1996, the *Journal of Bone and Joint Surgery (British)* published a 15.5-year study on whiplash-injured patients. The authors reported that 43% of these patients continued to suffer from clinically significant pain 15.5 years after injury. An additional 28% continued to suffer from nuisance pain at the 15.5-year analysis.

- In 2002, the *European Spine Journal* published a 17-year study on whiplash-injured patients. The authors reported that 55% of these patients continued to suffer from residual pain 17 years after injury. Of those with residual symptoms, 25% suffered from neck pain every day, and 23% had pain radiating into their arm daily.

- In 2006, the *Journal of Bone and Joint Surgery (British)* published a 30-year study on whiplash-injured patients. The authors reported that 15% of these patients continued to suffer from clinically significant pain 30 years after injury; their pain was such that they still required ongoing treatment. An additional 40% continued to suffer from nuisance pain at the 30-year analysis.